Aging Dogs Care

By

Dr. Stephanie Underwood

"Embracing the Golden Years: A Comprehensive Guide to Aged Dog Care" is an essential handbook for pet owners navigating the unique challenges of caring for senior dogs. This book delves into practical tips, nutritional insights, and holistic approaches to promote the well-being of aging canine companions. From understanding age-related health issues to creating a tailored care plan, this guide empowers readers to provide comfort, enhance quality of life, and forge a deeper, enduring bond with their cherished senior dogs."

Table of contents

Chapter 1

Understanding the Aging Process in Dogs

Understanding the aging process in dogs is crucial for responsible pet ownership and ensuring the well-being of our canine companions. Like humans, dogs go through distinct life stages, and as they age, their needs, behavior, and health requirements change. Here's an extensive overview of the aging process in dogs:

Puppyhood (0-1 year):

Puppyhood is a crucial developmental stage in a dog's life, typically spanning from birth to around one year of age, though the exact duration can vary by breed. This period is marked by rapid physical and behavioral changes as puppies transition from helpless newborns to more independent juveniles.

1. Neonatal Stage (0-2 Weeks): During the first two weeks, puppies are entirely dependent on their mother. They are blind, deaf, and unable to regulate their body temperature. Nursing and sleeping are primary

activities, and the mother provides essential care, including cleaning and feeding.

2. Transitional Stage (2-4 Weeks): Puppies begin to open their eyes, ears, and start developing motor skills. This is when they become more aware of their surroundings and start interacting with littermates. Socialization with siblings becomes crucial for later behavioral development.

3. Socialization Period (3-14 Weeks): A critical phase where puppies are highly impressionable. They learn from their experiences and should be exposed to various stimuli, people, environments, and other animals. Positive socialization during this time contributes to a well-adjusted adult dog.

4. Juvenile Stage (3-6 Months): Teething begins, and puppies often exhibit chewing behavior. Basic training can start during this period, and they may experience a fear period where new situations can be intimidating. Consistent, positive reinforcement helps shape their behavior.

5. Adolescence (6-12 Months): Growth continues, and sexual maturity may start, especially in larger breeds. Behavioral challenges, such as increased independence and testing boundaries, can arise. Obedience training remains important, and reinforcement of good behavior is crucial.

Key Aspects:

Healthcare: Regular veterinary check-ups, vaccinations, and a proper diet are vital for a healthy puppyhood.

Training: Basic commands, housebreaking, and socialization form the foundation for a well-behaved adult dog.

Nutrition: Puppies require a balanced diet rich in nutrients to support their rapid growth and development.

Play and Exercise: Play is essential for physical and mental stimulation. Gradual exposure to various environments and surfaces helps build confidence.

Successful navigation through puppyhood sets the stage for a well-adjusted and obedient adult dog. Owners play a pivotal role in providing a supportive and stimulating environment, ensuring a positive foundation for a lifelong bond.

Adulthood (1-7 years):

Adulthood in dogs is generally considered to begin around one to two years of age, depending on the breed. This phase varies between small and large breeds, with smaller dogs maturing more quickly. Here are some key aspects to understand about adulthood in dogs:

Physical Maturity:

Size and Growth: Dogs typically reach their full size during adulthood, with small breeds achieving maturity faster than larger ones.

Reproductive Maturity: Female dogs usually reach sexual maturity by their first heat cycle, while males may start exhibiting mating behaviors.

Behavioral Changes:

Energy Levels: Adult dogs generally have a more consistent energy level than puppies and may require regular exercise to maintain their health.

Social Behavior: Dogs often become more independent during adulthood, but their social nature persists, making ongoing socialization important.

Nutritional Needs:

Dietary Changes: As dogs mature, their nutritional requirements change. Transitioning to adult dog food is essential to support their energy levels and overall health.

Health Considerations:

Preventive Care: Regular veterinary check-ups become crucial to monitor for potential health issues, and vaccinations may need to be updated.

Dental Health: Adult dogs may require dental care to prevent issues like tartar buildup and gum disease.

Training and Obedience:

Continued Training: While basic training often starts during puppyhood, it's essential to maintain consistent training throughout adulthood to reinforce good behavior.

Life Expectancy:

Breed Variations: Different breeds have varying lifespans, with smaller breeds generally living longer than larger ones. However, individual factors such as genetics and overall care also play a role.

Senior Transition:

Onset of Aging: As dogs age, typically around 7 to 10 years, they enter the senior phase, and adjustments to diet, exercise, and veterinary care may be needed.

Understanding the various aspects of adulthood in dogs helps pet owners provide appropriate care and support tailored to their furry companions' changing needs. Regular attention to health, training, and overall well-being contributes to a fulfilling life for the adult dog.

Senior Years (7+ years):

Senior years in dogs, typically considered to begin around the age of 7, bring about significant changes in their health and behavior. One of the most noticeable transformations is the slowing down of their metabolism and energy levels. As dogs age, their activity levels often decrease, and they may become more prone to weight gain. It's crucial for owners to adjust their pet's diet accordingly, opting for senior-specific dog food to meet their changing nutritional needs.

Joint issues are a common concern in senior dogs, as the wear and tear on their joints over the years can lead to arthritis or other mobility issues. Providing supplements such as glucosamine and omega-3 fatty acids can aid in maintaining joint health and alleviate discomfort.

Dental care becomes increasingly important during the senior years. Dental problems, if left unaddressed, can lead to various health issues. Regular dental check-ups and appropriate chew toys can help keep their teeth clean and gums healthy.

Cognitive changes are also observed in senior dogs. Cognitive dysfunction syndrome (similar to Alzheimer's in humans) can manifest as disorientation, changes in sleep patterns, and altered behavior. Mental stimulation, interactive toys, and maintaining a consistent routine can contribute to cognitive health.

Regular veterinary check-ups become crucial in senior years to detect and manage potential health issues early. Bloodwork, urine analysis, and other diagnostic tests can help monitor organ function, identify any underlying diseases, and ensure proactive care.

Adjusting the living environment is essential. Senior dogs may benefit from softer bedding to support achy joints and ramps or steps to facilitate access to elevated surfaces. Additionally, maintaining a comfortable temperature is crucial for their overall well-being.

While physical activity decreases, mental stimulation remains vital. Engaging in gentle play, introducing new toys, and incorporating short walks can contribute to mental and emotional health. Senior dogs still crave social interaction and companionship.

Patience and understanding from owners are key during this life stage. Changes in behavior, such as increased clinginess or irritability, may occur, and it's essential to approach these shifts with empathy. Regular grooming and attention to skin and coat health also play a role in their overall comfort.

The senior years in dogs bring about various changes that require attentive and specialized care. With proper nutrition, veterinary attention, and a supportive environment, owners can ensure their senior dogs lead comfortable and fulfilling lives in their golden years.

Chapter 2

Signs of Aging Dogs

Signs of aging in dogs can vary depending on factors like breed, size, and overall health, but there are common indicators that may suggest your furry companion is entering their senior years:

Changes in Physical Appearance:

- Graying of the fur around the muzzle and eyes.

- Thinning of the coat and a duller appearance.

- Loss of muscle mass, leading to a more pronounced bony structure.

Alterations in Activity Levels:

- Reduced energy and enthusiasm for exercise.

- Reluctance to engage in strenuous activities or play.

- Slower movement and an overall decrease in agility.

Changes in Behavior:

- Increased sleep duration and frequency.

- Altered sleep patterns, such as more daytime napping.

- Changes in interaction with family members or other pets.

Cognitive Changes:

- Disorientation or confusion, especially in familiar surroundings.

- Forgetfulness or difficulty remembering commands.

- Reduced responsiveness to stimuli.

Dental Issues:

- Dental problems, including tooth decay and gum disease.

- Changes in eating habits due to oral discomfort.

Joint and Mobility Issues:

- Stiffness, especially after periods of rest.

- Difficulty climbing stairs or getting up from a lying position.

- Slower gait and a more cautious approach to physical activities.

Changes in Appetite and Weight:

- Changes in eating habits, such as reduced appetite or increased pickiness.

- Weight gain or loss, which may indicate changes in metabolism.

Organ Function Decline:

- Decreased kidney and liver function, leading to potential issues like increased thirst and changes in urine production.

- Changes in vision or hearing.

Incontinence:

- Difficulty controlling bladder or bowel movements.

Increased Susceptibility to Illness:

- Weakened immune system, making the dog more vulnerable to infections.

- Slower recovery from illnesses or injuries.

It's crucial to note that these signs can be indicative of various health issues, and not all aging dogs will display the same symptoms. Regular veterinary check-ups become especially important in the senior years to catch and address potential health concerns early. Additionally, a well-balanced diet, appropriate exercise, and mental stimulation can contribute to maintaining the overall well-being of an aging dog.

Chapter 3

Nutrition and Diet for Senior Dogs

Senior dogs have unique nutritional needs that should be addressed to ensure they lead healthy and happy lives. As dogs age, their metabolism, immune system, and energy levels change, necessitating adjustments in their diet. Here's an extensive overview of nutrition and diet considerations for senior dogs:

1. Protein:

Importance: Protein is vital for maintaining muscle mass, supporting the immune system, and overall body function.

Recommended Levels: Senior dogs may benefit from slightly higher protein levels than adult dogs to counteract muscle loss. However, individual needs vary, and consulting with a veterinarian is essential.

2. Fat:

Healthy Fats: Provide omega-3 and omega-6 fatty acids for joint health, cognitive function, and a shiny coat.

Moderation: While fat is essential, senior dogs are often less active, so it's crucial to monitor fat intake to prevent obesity.

3. Caloric Intake:

Adjustments: Senior dogs may require fewer calories, especially if they are less active. However, this varies depending on the dog's health, size, and activity level.

4. Fiber:

Digestive Health: Adequate fiber aids in digestion and helps prevent constipation, a common issue in older dogs.

Source: Look for easily digestible sources of fiber, such as sweet potatoes or pumpkin.

5. Joint Health:

Glucosamine and Chondroitin: Supplements like glucosamine and chondroitin can support joint health and mobility.

Omega-3 Fatty Acids: Reduce inflammation and promote joint comfort.

6. Dental Health:

Dental-Friendly Diets: Consider kibble size and texture that helps maintain dental health.

Regular Dental Check-ups: Senior dogs may be prone to dental issues, so regular veterinary dental check-ups are crucial.

7. Hydration:

Importance: Older dogs may be prone to dehydration, so ensure access to fresh water at all times.

Wet Food: Adding wet food to their diet can contribute to overall hydration.

8. Special Dietary Requirements:

Medical Conditions: Some senior dogs may have medical conditions that require specialized diets, such as kidney disease or diabetes. Consult with a vet for tailored recommendations.

9. Regular Veterinary Check-ups:

Monitoring Health: Regular check-ups allow veterinarians to monitor weight, assess overall health, and make necessary dietary adjustments.

10. Transitioning Diets:

Gradual Changes: When transitioning to a senior dog diet, do it gradually over a week to avoid digestive upset.

11. Quality Ingredients:

Premium Quality: Opt for high-quality dog food with easily digestible ingredients and minimal fillers.

12. Individualized Approach:

Tailored Plans: Each senior dog is unique, so consider individual factors like breed, size, health conditions, and activity level when creating a nutrition plan.

Meeting the nutritional needs of senior dogs requires a combination of quality ingredients, balanced nutrients, and a personalized approach.

Regular veterinary consultations play a crucial role in adjusting the diet to address specific age-related concerns and maintain optimal health.

Chapter 4

Exercise and Physical Activity for Senior Dogs

Regular exercise and physical activity play a crucial role in maintaining the health and well-being of senior dogs. As dogs age, their activity levels may naturally decrease, but it is essential to ensure that they still engage in appropriate exercise to prevent various health issues and promote a higher quality of life.

Tailored Exercise Routine:

Consult with your veterinarian to create a customized exercise plan based on your senior dog's breed, size, health condition, and overall fitness level.

Low-impact activities such as walking, swimming, and gentle play are excellent choices. These exercises are easier on aging joints and help maintain muscle tone.

Moderation is Key:

Be mindful of your senior dog's limitations. While exercise is vital, overexertion can lead to fatigue and potential injury.

Shorter, more frequent walks may be more suitable than longer sessions. Adjust the intensity and duration based on your dog's response.

Joint Health:

Senior dogs are prone to arthritis and joint issues. Incorporate exercises that promote joint flexibility, such as gentle stretching and controlled movements.

Consider joint supplements or specialized diets that support joint health, as recommended by your veterinarian.

Mental Stimulation:

Physical activity is not just about the body; it also stimulates the mind. Engage your senior dog in activities that challenge their cognitive abilities, such as puzzle toys and interactive games.

Weight Management:

Obesity is a common concern in senior dogs and can exacerbate joint problems. Regular exercise helps manage weight and contributes to overall health.

Adjust your senior dog's diet as needed and ensure they are receiving a well-balanced nutrition plan.

Regular Veterinary Check-ups:

Schedule regular veterinary check-ups to monitor your senior dog's health. Your vet can identify any emerging issues and adjust the exercise plan accordingly.

Socialization:

Maintain social interactions for mental well-being. Controlled playdates with compatible dogs or supervised group activities can provide both exercise and social stimulation.

Adapt the Environment:

Make your home environment senior-dog friendly. Use ramps or steps to help them navigate elevated surfaces, and provide soft bedding to support aging joints.

Hydration and Rest:

Ensure your senior dog stays well-hydrated, especially during physical activity. Provide opportunities for rest and recovery as needed.

Monitoring Behavior:

Pay attention to changes in behavior, such as limping, stiffness, or reluctance to exercise. These signs may indicate discomfort or pain, and prompt veterinary attention is essential.

In summary, a well-thought-out exercise and physical activity plan, coupled with attentive care and regular veterinary check-ups, can greatly contribute to the health and happiness of senior dogs. Always tailor activities to the individual needs of your furry companion, and make adjustments as they age to ensure they lead a fulfilling and comfortable life.

Chapter 5

Grooming and Skin care for aging dogs

As dogs age, grooming and skin care become crucial to ensure their well-being. Brush your dog regularly to remove loose fur and prevent matting, which can be uncomfortable for older dogs with sensitive skin. Use a gentle shampoo specifically formulated for senior dogs to avoid drying out their skin.

Check your dog's ears regularly for wax buildup or signs of infection. Trim their nails to a comfortable length, as overgrown nails can be painful for older dogs. Keep an eye on dental health by providing appropriate chew toys or dental treats, and consider regular teeth cleaning.

Moisturize your dog's skin with a pet-safe moisturizer, as aging skin tends to be more prone to dryness. Pay attention to any lumps, bumps, or changes in the skin, and consult your vet if you notice anything unusual.

Remember that grooming sessions also provide an opportunity to examine your aging dog for any potential health issues. Regular care and attention contribute to the overall comfort and health of your senior canine companion.

Chapter 6

Managing Chronic Conditions

Arthritis: Provide joint supplements, maintain a healthy weight, and consider anti-inflammatory medications prescribed by a vet.

Dental Issues: Regular dental care, including brushing and dental treats, can help manage dental problems in older dogs.

Cognitive Dysfunction Syndrome: Stimulate the mind with puzzles, maintain a routine, and consult your vet for possible medications.

Heart Disease: Administer prescribed medications, monitor for signs of heart failure, and maintain a low-sodium diet.

Diabetes: Consistent insulin therapy, a controlled diet, and regular exercise are essential in managing diabetes in dogs.

Kidney Disease: Specialized kidney diets, increased water intake, and regular vet check-ups are crucial for managing kidney issues.

Hypothyroidism: Daily medication as prescribed by the vet is necessary to manage thyroid hormone levels.

Cancer: Treatment options vary; consult with a veterinarian for appropriate therapies, which may include surgery, chemotherapy, or radiation.

Obesity: Control calorie intake, provide regular exercise, and monitor weight to prevent or manage obesity-related issues.

Hearing/Vision Loss: Create a safe environment, use hand signals for commands, and provide extra attention and care.

Always consult with a veterinarian for an accurate diagnosis and tailored management plan for your dog's specific condition. Regular veterinary check-ups are crucial for early detection and effective management of chronic conditions in aging dogs.

Chapter 7

Creating a Comfortable Living Environment for Aged Dogs

To create a comfortable living environment for aged dogs, consider these tips:

Orthopedic Bedding: Provide a soft and supportive bed to ease joint pain and arthritis.

Accessible Water: Ensure easy access to fresh water to keep them hydrated.

Gentle Exercise: Incorporate low-impact exercises to maintain mobility without straining joints.

Warmth: Keep the living space warm, as older dogs may be more sensitive to temperature changes.

Routine Vet Check-ups: Regular veterinary visits can address age-related health issues promptly.

Quality Nutrition: Feed a balanced diet suitable for their age and health requirements.

Non-Slip Flooring: Use rugs or mats to prevent slipping, especially on smooth surfaces.

Easy-to-Reach Essentials: Place food, water bowls, and toys at a height that doesn't require excessive bending.

Quiet Spaces: Provide a quiet, comfortable area where your dog can retreat for relaxation.

Regular Grooming: Maintain their coat and nails to prevent discomfort and hygiene issues.

Stimulating Toys: Offer toys that engage their mind without causing physical strain.

Consideration for Sensory Changes: Older dogs may experience hearing or vision loss, so be mindful of their surroundings.

Remember, individual needs may vary, and observing your dog's behavior will help tailor the environment to their specific comfort.

Chapter 8

End-of-Life Care and Decision-Making in Aged Dogs

End-of-life care for aged dogs involves a thoughtful and compassionate approach to ensure the comfort and well-being of the animal during their final stages. Decision-making during this period is crucial and often revolves around medical considerations, quality of life, and the emotional bond between the pet and their owner.

Assessment of Health Status:

Regular veterinary check-ups become crucial as dogs age. These visits help in assessing the overall health and detecting any chronic or terminal illnesses.

Diagnostic tests, such as blood work and imaging, may be recommended to evaluate the extent of the health issues.

Pain Management:

Identifying and managing pain is a key aspect of end-of-life care. Medications and alternative therapies can be employed to alleviate discomfort and improve the dog's quality of life.

Nutrition and Hydration:

Adjusting the dog's diet to meet their changing nutritional needs is essential. Some dogs may have decreased appetite, and providing palatable and easily digestible meals becomes important.

Ensuring proper hydration is crucial, especially if the dog is experiencing difficulties in eating or drinking.

Comfort and Environment:

Creating a comfortable and stress-free environment is vital. This may include providing a soft bed, warmth, and minimizing environmental stressors.

Paying attention to the dog's behavior and adjusting the surroundings accordingly helps in promoting a sense of security.

Communication with the Veterinarian:

Open communication with the veterinarian is essential throughout the process. Discussing the prognosis, treatment options, and expected outcomes helps in making informed decisions.

Quality of Life Considerations:

Assessing the dog's quality of life involves monitoring their daily activities, appetite, and overall happiness. This evaluation helps in determining when the dog may be experiencing more discomfort than joy.

Family and Emotional Support:

Owners often experience emotional challenges during this time. Providing emotional support to both the dog and the owner is crucial. This may include spending quality time with the pet and seeking counseling if needed.

Advance Care Planning:

Discussing and planning for end-of-life decisions in advance can be beneficial. This may involve determining preferences for euthanasia, burial, or cremation.

Euthanasia:

Making the decision for euthanasia is one of the most difficult aspects of end-of-life care. It is typically considered when the dog's suffering becomes unbearable, and medical intervention cannot provide a reasonable quality of life.

Aftercare:

Planning for aftercare, including burial or cremation, is another consideration. Some owners may choose to keep a memorial or perform a small ceremony to honor their pet's memory.

In summary, end-of-life care for aged dogs involves a holistic approach that considers medical, emotional, and ethical aspects. Regular communication with a veterinarian, assessing the dog's well-being, and providing support for both the pet and the owner are crucial components of this process.

Chapter 9:

List of 100 Dog Breeds and their Average Life Expectancies.

List 100 dog breeds and their Average life expectancies

1. Affenpinscher - 12 to 15 years

2. Afghan Hound - 12 to 15 years

3. Airedale Terrier - 10 to 13 years

4. Alaskan Malamute - 10 to 14 years

5. American Eskimo Dog - 12 to 16 years

6. American Water Spaniel - 10 to 14 years

7. Anatolian Shepherd Dog - 10 to 13 years

8. Australian Cattle Dog - 12 to 16 years

9. Australian Shepherd - 12 to 15 years

10.   Basenji - 12 to 16 years

11.   Beagle - 10 to 15 years

12.   Belgian Tervuren - 10 to 12 years

13.   Bernese Mountain Dog - 6 to 8 years

14.   Bichon Frise - 12 to 15 years

15.   Black Russian Terrier - 10 to 14 years

16.   Bolognese - 12 to 14 years

17.   Border Collie - 12 to 16 years

18.   Borzoi - 10 to 12 years

19.   Boston Terrier - 11 to 13 years

20.   Boxer - 9 to 12 years

21.   Bull Terrier - 10 to 14 years

22.   Bulldog - 8 to 12 years

23.   Bullmastiff - 8 to 10 years

24.   Cairn Terrier - 12 to 16 years

25.   Cavalier King Charles Spaniel - 9 to 14 years

26.   Chesapeake Bay Retriever - 10 to 13 years

27.   Chihuahua - 12 to 20 years

28.   Clumber Spaniel - 10 to 12 years

29.   Cocker Spaniel - 10 to 14 years

30.   Dachshund - 12 to 16 years

31.   Dachshund (Miniature) - 12 to 16 years

32.   Dalmatian - 10 to 13 years

33.   Doberman Pinscher - 10 to 13 years

34.   Entlebucher Mountain Dog - 10 to 15 years

35.   Eskimo Dog - 12 to 15 years

36.   Finnish Lapphund - 12 to 15 years

37.   French Bulldog - 10 to 12 years

38.   German Shepherd - 9 to 13 years

39.   Golden Retriever - 10 to 12 years

40.   Great Dane - 7 to 10 years

41.   Great Pyrenees - 10 to 12 years

42.   Greyhound - 10 to 14 years

43.   Harrier - 10 to 12 years

44.   Havanese - 13 to 15 years

45.   Icelandic Sheepdog - 12 to 15 years

46.   Irish Water Spaniel - 10 to 12 years

47.   Irish Wolfhound - 6 to 8 years

48.   Italian Greyhound - 12 to 15 years

49.   Japanese Chin - 10 to 12 years

50.   Keeshond - 12 to 15 years

51.   Komondor - 10 to 12 years

52.   Labrador Retriever - 10 to 14 years

53.   Leonberger - 8 to 10 years

54. Lhasa Apso - 12 to 15 years

55. Lowchen - 12 to 14 years

56. Maltese - 12 to 15 years

57. Manchester Terrier - 14 to 16 years

58. Mastiff - 6 to 10 years

59. Miniature Schnauzer - 12 to 15 years

60. Newfoundland - 9 to 10 years

61. Norfolk Terrier - 12 to 15 years

62. Norwegian Buhund - 12 to 15 years

63. Nova Scotia Duck Tolling Retriever - 12 to 14 years

64. Papillon - 13 to 16 years

65. Papillon - 13 to 16 years

66. Pembroke Welsh Corgi - 12 to 15 years

67. Pharaoh Hound - 12 to 14 years

68.   Plott Hound - 12 to 14 years

69.   Polish Lowland Sheepdog - 12 to 15 years

70.   Pomeranian - 12 to 16 years

71.   Poodle - 10 to 15 years

72.   Portuguese Water Dog - 10 to 14 years

73.   Pug - 12 to 15 years

74.   Redbone Coonhound - 10 to 12 years

75.   Rottweiler - 8 to 10 years

76.   Saint Bernard - 8 to 10 years

77.   Saluki - 12 to 14 years

78.   Samoyed - 12 to 14 years

79.   Scottish Terrier - 11 to 13 years

80.   Shetland Sheepdog - 12 to 14 years

81.   Shetland Sheepdog - 12 to 14 years

82.   Shiba Inu - 13 to 16 years

83.   Shih Tzu - 10 to 18 years

84.   Shih Tzu - 10 to 18 years

85.   Shiloh Shepherd - 9 to 14 years

86.   Siberian Husky - 12 to 15 years

87.   Silky Terrier - 12 to 15 years

88.   Staffordshire Bull Terrier - 12 to 16 years

89.   Sussex Spaniel - 10 to 12 years

90.   Tibetan Mastiff - 10 to 14 years

91.   Tibetan Spaniel - 12 to 15 years

92.   Tibetan Terrier - 12 to 15 years

93.   Tibetan Terrier - 12 to 15 years

94.   Toy Fox Terrier - 12 to 15 years

95.   Vizsla - 10 to 14 years

96.   Weimaraner - 10 to 13 years

97.   West Highland White Terrier - 13 to 16 years

98.   Wire Fox Terrier - 13 to 15 years

99.   Xoloitzcuintli - 12 to 14 years

100.   Yorkshire Terrier - 11 to 15 years